Jogging and Running Guide: The Benefits of

The Best Jogging and Running Guide for Beginners

By: Steven Stewart

9781634286848

NPL F

Nashville Public Library   FOUNDATION

Books and other materials
on Healthcare
made possible
through the generosity of
St. Thomas Hospital

NPLF.ORG

PUBLISHERS NOTES

Disclaimer – Speedy Publishing LLC

This book was originally printed before 2014. This is an adapted reprint by Speedy Publishing LLC with newly updated content designed to help readers with much more accurate and timely information and data.

Speedy Publishing LLC

40 E Main Street, Newark, Delaware, 19711

Contact Us: 1-888-248-4521

Website: http://www.speedypublishing.co

REPRINTED Paperback Edition: ISBN: 9781634286848

Manufactured in the United States of America

DEDICATION

I dedicate this book to my brother, Allen. We both know how difficult it is to have an unhealthy lifestyle. Thank you bro for always being there for me.

TABLE OF CONTENTS

Publishers Notes.. 2

Dedication 3

Table of Contents... 4

Chapter 1- Jogging and Running – Doing it Right 5

Chapter 2- Have Jogging into Your System........................13

Chapter 3- Tips on How to Properly Jog...........................19

Chapter 4- Listen to Your Body When Jogging..................27

Chapter 5- Jog, Sprint and Marathon for Easy Weight Loss 39

Chapter 6- Doing your Marathon Right.............................46

Chapter 7- Cycling is Another Way to Do it.......................51

Chapter 8- Cycling as a Recreational Activity....................57

Chapter 9- Panoramic View and Extreme Weight Loss.................68

Chapter 10- Losing Weight with Your Friends 75

About The Author..87

CHAPTER 1- JOGGING AND RUNNING – DOING IT RIGHT

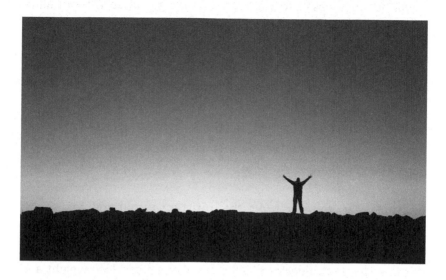

Jogging to Lose Weight

Anyone who is trying to lose weight needs to engage in some kind of aerobic exercise in order to boost the metabolism to burn calories faster. Although a brisk walk will suffice, many people are more comfortable with jogging and feel it works better for them.

Making the choice to jog during weight loss will not only help you lose weight but will also help you get into the routine of exercising, a move that will help you keep the weight off when you have reached your goal weight. The ideal exercise for weight loss is a combination of aerobic and resistance exercise—jogging combined with some weight lifting routines.

Getting into the habit of jogging is not a difficult one for most people, but if you have never been one to exercise, it may come as a shock at first. You do not want to try to jump right into a long jogging workout but rather begin slowly and work your way up to where you want to be. Do not rush to reach the amount of time you wish to spend jogging but let your body guide you and let you know when you are ready. If you allow your body to be your guide, it will be much easier to work into a jogging routine without all of the discomfort.

In order to achieve the ultimate weight loss, you want to make jogging part of your routine but not the only exercise you perform. Although aerobic exercise is what helps you burn calories, resistance exercise helps you build lean muscle mass which burns fan faster. Therefore the perfect routine is a combination of aerobic and resistance exercise.

Of course, if you can't do the resistance routines for health reasons, then certainly you can obtain the benefits from jogging but you may find it takes longer to accomplish. However, any kind of exercise you can perform will certainly help you lose weight and keep it off after you have reached your goal weight. You have to remember you will need to keep it up in order to maintain your weight loss. You cannot stop once you have reached your goal weight and expect to maintain the results.

Do not overdo your jogging in an attempt to lose weight faster. Though you may accomplish that goal, it will be at the cost of your health. Working your muscles too hard even in jogging can cause your muscles and cartilage to become damaged thus preventing you from doing many activities including jogging.

Choose a Jogging Trail that is Away from Traffic

Although you want to job in places that are well populated you also want to stay away from traffic. Do not choose high traffic roads to jog even if you are on the side of the road facing traffic. There is always the possible that a car or truck will veer off the road and hit you or maybe just pull off the road with mechanical problems and fail to see you. If you choose roads that have a high traffic volume, choose one that has a sidewalk or a shoulder that is far enough off the main road for you to be safe.

In addition to the potential for being hit jogging in a high traffic area, is the possibility of being mugged or even kidnapped as you jog alongside the road. You can avoid those possibilities by making sure you are on the sidewalk or far enough away from the highway that someone would have to stop the car and get out in order to pull you into the car. Safety is a very important issue for joggers and one that you should not take lightly. Jogging is a healthy activity for the body but you also have to make sure you perform it with your personal safety in mind.

One of the best ways to make certain you are in a well-lit area that is well populated is in a business area. Keep in mind that not all business sections will follow this pattern, so you still have to be careful where you go. For example, factories and warehouses are not the safest places to be because even though people may be working, they are usually secluded and unable to see what is going on outside. The best places are round stores where customers come and go at all times rather than restaurants or movie theaters where customers are frequently inside rather than outside.

The key to making jogging a healthy activity is to make certain you are aware of the surroundings where you jog and to be attentive to your surroundings. Do not make yourself a target by being preoccupied with your own thoughts or with a music player. Although it may help pass the time while you are jogging it also puts your safety in danger and makes you vulnerable to a surprise attack by someone you neither saw nor heard.

One of the most important things to consider when jogging is your clothing, especially the type of shoes you wear. You want something that is comfortable and that is specifically for running or jogging. You can also choose cross trainers if you desire, but it is better to have something with cushioning such as the Nike Air and similar shoes.

The cushioning in the shoes will help prevent any hard landing on your feet as well as allowing airflow through your feet to prevent damage to the feet, knees and legs. If you have to make sacrifices due to budgetary concerns do not do it with your shoes. The shoes are the most important part of your jogging clothing when it comes to preventing injury.

Your outer clothing is also important because you do not want to be too cold or too warm. In the warmer months, you can certainly choose shorts and a short sleeve or sleeveless top or shirt, but you also want to make sure, if you are jogging during the daylight hours to protect your skin from the sun with sun block that has an SPF of at least 15.

You also want to wear a sun hat or cap that protects your head and prevents heat stroke or heat exhaustion. During colder months, you will want to choose, either sweat pants or track pants. Never go out jogging wearing short sleeves when it is cold outside. You may feel you will stay warm because of your exercise but the reality is that the sweat from your body mingling with the cold air makes a perfect environment for illness.

If you are going jogging during a time when there is likely to be a severe change in temperature you may want to take along a light jacket and tie it around your waist while you are jogging. In the event the temperature drops substantially you will be able to put your jacket on and shield yourself from the cold. Use a waist pack to carry any money or keys you need rather than attempting to carry even a small purse that a mugger can easily take. Better yet, put your money and keys in your pocket where they are out of view from people. The less opportunity you provide for criminal acts the least likely you are to become a victim.

Choosing Well Lit Places to Jog

Jogging may be your exercise of choice but you also want to make sure you exercise precautions when you job. This is especially important for women although men are certainly not immune to acts of violence. One of the most important things to remember is to always job in well-lit areas. If you go to a park, stay away from any areas that are secluded such as bushes and trees. You want to choose well-lit areas so you can see what is going on and are on the lookout for any strangers and anyone who looks suspicious.

If the area where you customarily jog does not have, lights avoid that area or take your own. You never want to take the chance of someone jumping at you suddenly and you are not able to see the person. No matter where you live you do not want to take a chance— even, high-class neighborhoods have criminals or criminals come in from other areas. You do not want to take a chance of being another statistic because you failed to exercise reasonable precautions by making sure to job in a well-lit area.

Besides avoiding criminal activity, it is also a good idea to jog in a well-lit area so that you are able to follow the trail you have set for yourself. If you are jogging after dark, it is very easy to lose track of where you are going, especially if you are concentrating more on your jog than on where you are going. Certainly, it is preferable to job while it is still light, but if that is not possible because of work commitments or other valid reason, make sure you can see where you are going and who might be hiding in the shadows.

The best rule to follow when jogging is to exercise caution and know where you are going. Never choose areas you do not know even if they are well lit and appear to be populated. Nighttime is not the time to learn new places to go or attempt to decide if an area is bright enough for you to see anyone who may come out from the shadows. There are many would-be attackers that are looking for those who have failed to exercise precautions and are therefore very vulnerable and an easy prey. Do not be one of the unlucky ones.

Creating Your Own Jogging Trail

For those who live in rural areas or even suburban areas with a good deal of land, you might want to consider creating your own jogging trail. It does not have to be anything fancy, and you can choose to use grass or dirt at your preference. Some people may even find it helpful to use AstroTurf or a similar product—"fake grass" instead of the real thing. The choice you make is yours but you want to make sure the design and space meets your needs. Check it before you begin so that you make sure you allow enough space because once you finish there is no going back without redoing the entire jogging trail.

Another possibility for those who live in a neighborhood with a lot of open land is to obtain permission to create a jogging trail on a piece of that open land. In many cases, the open land belongs to the state or the county, and for a good cause, they may even do the construction and foot the cost for you if enough people are interested. Even if they will not finance the project, all you need is permission to use the land for the jogging trail. It is something that would be a benefit to the community as a whole much as a park is beneficial to the children of a community.

Sometimes it is not necessary to obtain permission to create a jogging trail; it depends where you want to place it. Certainly if it is part of your property, you will not need permission as long as you stay within the bounds of your own property and do not create any obstructions that would prevent public access to water or sewer lines. A project would not only be beneficial but inexpensive.

Having your own jogging trail would also mean you do not have to worry about your safety in a remote area and would make the activity more enjoyable for you. In addition, you would never have to worry about going out in the weather or wondering where you could go to jog.

If you are considering creating your own jogging trail, you might want to get together with a neighbor and perhaps build one the two of you can share. This project can be a benefit to more than one person and would help both families become healthier by engaging in a mutual exercise.

Developing a Jogging Routine

Before you begin jogging, you want to develop a routine that combines jogging with walking or running. Although jogging is fine in itself, a combination of other aerobic exercise is much better on the body.

Jogging is a good way to develop a slow and rhythmic pace but it can also be bad on the calves and knees if you are not careful. That is one reason it's better to try to combine jogging with running or walking. If possible, try to do your jogging on a soft—or at least smooth—surface. The softer the surface on which you jog the easier it will be on your legs. Of course, it can be difficult to jog on grass unless it is solid, so the time of year you are attempting to jog will have a huge impact on where you can jog.

You want to develop a routine that does not cause you to run the risk of injury. That means stopping when your body has told you that you have had enough. Even if you develop a routine that calls for one hour per day, let your knees and legs be the guide. If they are beginning to hurt, do not continue insisting you are going to meet your goals.

Continuing when you are experiencing pain can be detrimental to your health. The idea of jogging is to develop and participate in a healthy activity that allows you to burn calories and increase your heart rate. That does not mean you have to cause health problems for yourself in the meantime by any means. You can gradually build to a pace your body can tolerate—there is no need to do it all in one day or even a week. While some people may be able to develop a good routine in a week, it may take others a couple of weeks or even a month.

The level of tolerance for each person will be different which is why you cannot develop your routine based upon any general set of rules. You also cannot follow someone else's guidelines about how long you should jog or how long it should take you to be able to reach your ultimate goal. No two people are alike and you have to follow your own body and tolerances. If you attempt to push yourself beyond your body's tolerances, you will defeat the purpose of your jogging routine.

CHAPTER 2- HAVE JOGGING INTO YOUR SYSTEM

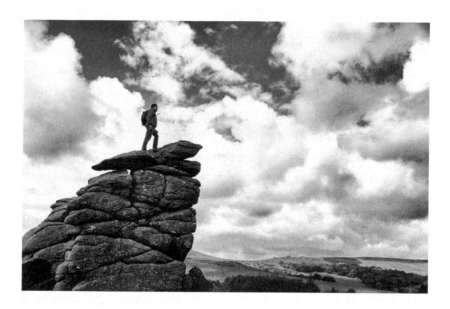

Don't Overdo it

Sometimes we are tempted to overdo things in the exercise department. With resistance exercises the worse you're going to do is have some sore muscles for a few days—in most cases anyway—but if you overdo it when you're jogging you run the risk of damaging your knees or calves.

The consistent pressure on the balls of the feet and the knees will eventually take a toll on those parts of your body if you are not careful. That means not to attempt to jog for hours at a time even if you may split it up throughout the day. You want to set aside perhaps an hour a day for jogging and only if you are able to do so.

When you first start jogging you want to begin slowly and gradually increase the amount of time you spend jogging. If you find your legs or knees are hurting stop jogging. Do not attempt to rest and go back later but stop for the day. When your body becomes used to the new routine you will then be able to spend more time jogging during the day—perhaps even stop when you begin to hurt and return later.

However, you do not want to attempt to do this until your body including your legs, knees and feet become used to jogging.

If you want to continue with your exercise routine when you knees and legs are beginning to hurt or tire, you might be able to resort to brisk walking rather than jogging. Walking will put less stress on your legs and knees and will be safer when you are no longer able to jog. Even walking at a leisurely pace is acceptable at this stage in order to prevent injury. The idea is to learn how to exercise on a regular basis, not wear out your body parts so that you are no longer able to do the things you are used to doing.

Jogging can be a fun and healthy activity if you make sure you let your body tell you when it has had enough. There is nothing any worse than continuing to exercise long after your body has told you it has had enough. Although you may set a period for your exercise, you want your body to be the final judge of when you have had enough for the day.

Dress for the Weather When Jogging

Although you want to dress so that you do not become overheated, you also want to dress for the weather. Even if you feel you will become sufficiently warm, do not go outside in cold weather wearing shorts and a tee shirt. The combination of the cold outside and your sweat from jogging will cause you to become chilled and creates the potential for illness. Instead, you want to wear a sweat suit or tracksuit during cold weather. You may feel you will be overly war but in reality, you will not become warm enough to justify wearing shorts in the middle of the winter.

Although you may be one of the people who is tempted to jog no matter what kind of weather you might encounter keep in mind that your purpose is to perform healthy exercise, and you cannot do that if you insist on jogging when there is snow, ice, sleet or freezing rain. That may sound like common sense, but if you look outside you will find at least one or two people jogging during extreme weather. Even in the summer months, it can be detrimental to your health to job in the rain because the combination of sweat and rain can still give you a chill and cause a summer cold.

The worst times to jog in terms of clothing are likely to be spring and fall because of the potential for a severe change in temperatures as the sun goes down. You need to be ready for these changes and not assume you can wear the same jogging outfit at any time of the day or evening. Always be aware of weather changes throughout the day and adjust your clothing accordingly. The inclination to wear shorts when you jog no matter what they weather may be is one that causes many people to become ill.

Use common sense and proceed with caution. Dress for the weather and do not go jogging if you are already sick. Although it may be a healthy activity, it can cause those with a low immune system to become very ill if they are not careful. Remember, it does not take much to break down your immune system—one of the easiest ways to do that is lack of sleep or general fatigue. In addition, activities such as smoking also wear on the immune system and make a person more susceptible to colds and other illnesses.

Is Jogging Healthy for Everyone?

Although jogging is a healthy form of exercise, it is definitely not for everyone. Some people have health conditions that prevent them from jogging such as knee problems or even heart problems. There are also those who have respiratory problems that may not want to participate in jogging, at least not during the summer when they are most likely to be overheated and possibly have an attack.

Although most people are physically able to jog, you should always check with your doctor if you have any physical condition that might make it unsafe. You want to make the right choice or jogging will not improve your health. In fact, if you undertake jogging when you have poor health it will defeat the purpose.

Anyone who is not able to do any kind of running or at least brisk walking should probably not participate in jogging. That also includes anyone who has back, knee or leg problems because the additional stress can possibly create more problems. That does not mean those people should not participate in any kind of exercise but they should choose something their doctor recommends and that will consider their condition. You do not want to create more health problems for yourself by participating in an activity that your body cannot handle.

The choice you make will allow you to continue living an active lifestyle but if you make the wrong choice, you are liable to find you are unable to do the same things you used to be able to do. It is important to know your limitations and accept them for what they are rather than trying to overcome them.

When we were young, we never let things get us down and made it a point to overcome any limitations that may have presented themselves. As we get older, we have to work around those limitations. That means you do not try to do things that you know are impossible or will cause injury to any body parts. That includes jogging and any other activities that you may no longer be able to perform. It is easy enough to find something else—brisk walking or leisurely walking for instance. There is no need to be stress on your body because you thought you could still jog about you had knee surgery. Be reasonable—there are enough activities for everyone who is interested in improving their health with aerobic exercise.

Is Jogging Safe for Heart Patients?

Although heart patients are encouraged to walk, is it safe for them to jog? After all, there is only minimal difference between brisk walking and jogging. The thing to remember is that different patients have different degrees of heart problems. It is important to remember that the cardiologist is the one who knows fully how serious a patient's condition is. While one patient may be perfect fine with jogging, another one may only allow brisk or even leisurely walking. The final answer falls under knowing how much stress an individual patient's heart can take based on the health of that patient only.

Regardless of how well you may feel, never undertake jogging without the permission of your doctor. There may be any number of reasons your doctor does not want you to jog, especially if you have undergone heart surgery. It takes time to heal, and only your doctor can determine at one point you are healed enough to participate in jogging. It is by far more strenuous than just walking, so you do not want to jog until and unless your doctor approves. An exercise that is as healthy as jogging is not necessarily healthy for everyone and thus may cause health problems rather than create a healthier body.

Jogging And Running Guide: The Benefits Of Running

What if your doctor does not tell you whether you can jog or not after a heart attack or heart surgery, like any diet or exercise routine, do you participate unless you consult your doctor first. You need to speak to your doctor and let him know the exercise routine you wish to perform, and he will let you know if you can do it. If he tells you no, you are free to question his reasons but under no circumstances should you make your own decision about it.

Remember, the doctor has all of your health records including EKGs, so you need to trust his best judgment. Even if he tells you that you are limited to walk leisurely for the rest of your life, you must accept that he is doing what is best for you.

Even if you have not had a heart attack but have a heart condition that may have an effect by jogging, always ask your doctor before you participate. Only your doctor knows the factors that may affect your heart condition and/or make it worse. Do not be fooled into thinking jogging is healthy for everyone because there are conditions under which hat may not be the case.

CHAPTER 3- TIPS ON HOW TO PROPERLY JOG

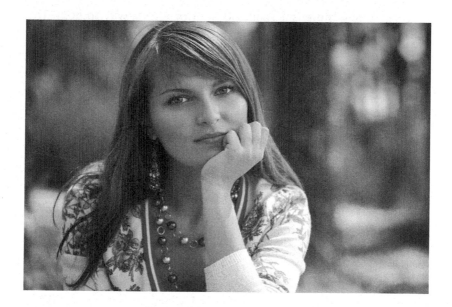

Good solid question, right, how do you jog? Is there a right or wrong way to jog? Although some might say it makes no difference, others may disagree with that. Everyone has his or her own personal preference about different things, and when those preferences are different from what others may do, it means the other person is "wrong." Is that actually true? No, it is not necessarily true, but in the eyes of the person doing things differently, it is indeed the wrong way of doing whatever activity it was.

Whether it is jogging, running, or even vacuuming the floor, some people believe there is a right and wrong way to do it.

In retrospect, jogging involves the slow, rhythmic movement of a run, more like a trot or gallop of a horse than an actual run. Because of its slower pace, people who cannot run can usually jog. That is not always the case; there are exceptions such as heart patients and others who may not have the ability to perform any activity beyond that of a brisk or leisurely walk. For those who have the pleasure of being able to jog, they will develop their own way of doing it, and there is actually no right or wrong way to do it. The key issue is being up to keep up a slow steady pace but there is no right or wrong way except in the minds of some perfectionists.

No matter what you teach people about jogging, they are still going to find their own methodology, something that works for them. The choice is personal and as long as the result is the same there is little relevance to the reasoning or methodology that separates one person's style from another.

There will always be different ways to jog based on a person's personal preference and even of their weight and body build. Some people just find one way of jogging easier than another with some even choosing to alternate between jogging and brisk walking and even running. It is not your style of jogging that will make a difference in your health but rather your perseverance in doing it. Choosing to remain healthy by participating in jogging as your exercise of choice will provide you with more years of good health than those who choose to lead a sedentary lifestyle.

Jogging and Walking: the Perfect Combination

If you enjoy both jogging and walking or maybe find you cannot jog for very long at a time, you might want to consider a combination of both. You can start out jogging and as you begin to tire or feel pain in your knees or legs, switch to brisk walking.

Many health professionals will even tell you that brisk walking is better for you than running, so substituting walking during your daily jog is not going to minimize the health benefits of jogging. In fact, you will find that you can increase the length of time you can participate when you combine the two activities instead of trying to jog o walk during the entire time.

One reason it is much more beneficial to combine jogging with walking is that each activity has certain limitations in terms of health benefits. For example, jogging too much can cause problems with your knees and calves while walking at a brisk pace may be too much for someone people to accomplish at one time. By combining the two activities, you can decrease the amount of time you participate thus making it easier on those who find it difficult to walk or jog for very long at one time.

Does that mean you can combine jogging with a leisurely walk? That depends on what you are expecting from the jog. A leisurely walk will provide some benefits but not as many as a brisk walk. A leisurely walk is not likely to increase your heart rate and thus will not provide the entire required amount of exercise a person needs on a daily basis. This is especially true for those who are walking or jogging along with a weight loss plan. In order to gain the benefits of aerobic exercises it is important to have a certain momentum along with speed. You might slow down your jog to a brisk walk but you do not want to turn it into a leisurely walk. If you want a leisurely walk, which is very good exercise as well, you want to do that at another time.

Being able to combine brisk walking with jogging with also help prevent some of the problems that are associated with jogging. Not everyone experiences any of those problems but if you already have calf or knee problems, you can minimize any future potential problems if you use the combination of walking and jogging.

Jogging or Running: What Difference Does it Make?

When it comes to exercise, does it really matter if you jog or if you run? Perhaps in theory, it does not make a difference but in reality, you are much better off with jogging. Why is that you may ask? When you run, you tend to begin fast, slow down or stop when you tire, then attempt to pick up speed again. The problem is that you have lost momentum by that time and most likely do not have the ability to regain the power you had in the beginning. You will therefore tire easier and take longer to recover your strength and momentum.

Jogging on the other hand allows you to maintain a slow pace from the start therefore, you are less likely to slow down and stop forcing you to lose your momentum. In that respect, you will be in a better position to not only benefit from the jogging itself, but also to be able to use it to boost the metabolic system so it can burn calories. That is not to say that you cannot accomplish it with running but the fact that you tend to slow down and stop more often while you are running makes it less desirable as an activity for burning calories. Running is good for exercising the legs but as a way to boost the metabolism and burn calories the slow but steady pace of jogging is much better.

Of course, some people prefer to engage in a combination of running and jogging and for them the effect is the same. Because you are still jogging you will be able to get the metabolism running while at the same time keeping up your momentum going with jogging. When you combine running and jogging, you have less of a tendency to slow completely down as you do with a steady run.

Therefore, you are able to keep the momentum at steadier pace though not as steady as it would be if you were only jogging. You can still gain many benefits from the combination of running and jogging, especially if you allow yourself to maintain timeliness and not just take a few minutes and quit. Build up to an hour a day and you will soon see a big difference in the way you feel in general, look and feel about yourself and your life.

Jogging, Running and Walking, the Aerobic Threesome

When it comes to aerobic exercise, jogging is only one of the three common ones. The combination of jogging, running and walking will go together to form a perfect threesome in the world of aerobic exercise. It is important to understand the importance of aerobic exercise with the most important being its ability to increase the body's metabolism thus making it easier to burn calories. That in itself is a condition for a healthy body since that means either the body will be able to maintain a healthy weight or help a dieter burn fat faster in order to burn more calories than he or she consumes.

Since the fat burners are the aerobic exercises, it makes sense that running, walking and jogging are the perfect combination. Being able to participate in all three throughout the day will make the job easier, especially if one participates in brisk walking as opposed to leisurely walking. Participating in these three aerobic exercises guarantees that you do not become tired or bored with any one activity and are able to continue working on your exercise routine. Of course, you can also add in skiing, bicycling and swimming in order to provide an all around group of fun aerobic exercises.

Choosing from several different exercises in addition to jogging can provide the perfect balance of exercise to boost the metabolism. Whether you are trying to just remain healthy or lose weight you still need to learn how to burn calories or you will gain weight. The body must burn calories that are equal to what you consume in order to maintain your weight or burn more than you consume in order to lose weight. That makes it difficult unless you do exercise that help the body burn those calories. Most people consider jogging to be a fun activity, but you also have to make sure you do it safely with properly fitting shoes and in a safe area.

Combining jogging, running and walking are a good combination for anyone wishing to either maintain or lose weight. You do not have to be on a diet to want to burn fat—you may just need to tone parts of your body. Jogging provides that as you swing your arms as you jog along your designated track or trail. The more rhythmic your movements are the more likely you are to burn more calories.

Will Jogging Make Bad Knees Worse?

You hear a great deal of information about jogging causing knee problems. What about those who already have knee problems, will it make them worse? Is there a way to prevent knee problems when you jog? One of the best ways to prevent knee problems when you jog is to make sure you wear the right kind of shoes. You do not want to go to the department store and buy some cheap street sneakers; you want to choose athletic shoes that have specific design for running. Some people prefer cross trainers that are for many different activities but when it comes to jogging, it might be better to choose a running shoe.

If you already have bad knees you may want to consider another activity. Jogging in itself can cause problems with your knees if you are not careful; therefore attempting to jog when you already have bad knees may be courting disaster. You want to protect your knees from any further damage by making sure you do not participate in any activity that will cause additional damage. For those with bad knees walking may be better than jogging because of the reduced stress on the knees. It might not be exactly what you want to do, but you have to decide between walking and causing additional damage to your knees. If you make the wrong choice you may end up having knee surgery with no guarantee the problem will correct permanently.

Most joggers who have knee problems developed knee problems after they began jogging. In many cases, it is because of the stress placed on the knees while jogging. In other cases, bad knees result from improper fitting shoes, especially from the era when sneakers were the only form of athletic wear that was available. There were no specially made athletic shoes for running, only for sports like football, basketball, baseball and golf. Running shoes is new on the market when compared to how long jogging and track have been activities.

Thus, many of the people who have knee problems related to jogging are older people who began jogging before running shoes were available or at least before people were aware of the importance of wearing running shoes. Today those people are suffering from knee and calf problems, many unable to even walk any more than around their homes and to the store.

Jogging Your Way to a Healthier You

Everyone needs to get into the routine of doing some kind of exercise in order to remain healthy. For some people, that involves developing a jogging routine while others may choose a different kind of exercise. Although jogging is not for everyone, some people are quite content with this activity. Unlike running, when you jog you are at a slower, rhythmic pace which makes it possible to jog for longer than you can run. Though some people are able to run at a slow gait, most people tend to begin running at a fast pace and slow down or stop when they get tired then pick up speed again.

That type of routine can tire you out quicker and prevent you from accomplishing everything you want to accomplish.

Before you begin jogging you want to decide where you want to jog, keeping in mind that you need to choose a safe and well-lit area that has a level and smooth surface. Once you know where you can jog with confidence, you can begin working on the routine you want to accomplish.

Keep in mind you want to start slowly and gradually build up to where you want to be. If you want to jog for an hour a day, do not attempt to begin with that but rather start slowly and build yourself to that level. At the same time, you do not want to push yourself to reach your goal in a week or two—let your body guide you and help you reach your final goal. There is no need to be in a hurry to reach your final goal; you have reached this point in your life without jogging so take it easy.

As you are working toward your final goal be realistic in your expectations. You might want to begin with fifteen minutes and increase it gradually. The idea is to reach your final goal, not to give yourself excruciating pain so that you cannot move. Being in pain from jogging is certainly not the way to begin enjoying this or any other activity. When you begin slowly so that you do not experience substantial pain, you will be more likely to want to continue jogging. Most people will not return to an activity that causes them pain on a regular basis. Gradually increasing the amount of time you spend jogging will help you reduce that possibility.

CHAPTER 4- LISTEN TO YOUR BODY WHEN JOGGING

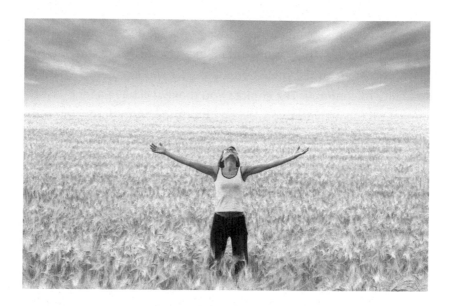

One of the most important things to remember about jogging is to let your body tell you when you have had enough. It does not matter if you have only been jogging for fifteen minutes; if your calves and knees are beginning to hurt, you need to stop for the day. You may think you will not experience any lasting effects if you continue but the truth is you can do severe damage to your knees and calves unless you list to your body. Even if you have been jogging for years, you need to stop if you begin to hurt because there may be a reason your body is sending your messages.

One problem that is adamant is that many people still want to live by the adage "no pain no gain,' but time has shown that if you abide by that premise you will do your body more harm than good. People have damaged their legs and knees beyond repair by continuing to exercise when they should have already stopped. You may think you are taking the easy way out, but in reality, you are protecting your body from further damage. Once you damage your muscles or cartilage and continue to exert pressure on that tissue, you run the risk of doing permanent damage.

Allowing your body to be your guide is not something you just do when you begin jogging but something you need to follow anything you participate in that or any other exercise activity. You need to allow your body to tell you when it has had enough and when it has to ability to continue. The choices you make will have a long-lasting impact on the activities you will be able to perform during your life and thus the decisions you make regarding your jogging routines should take all of this into consideration. You only get one body and therefore you need to take care not to damage any of its internal components including muscles, bones and cartilage.

Another mistake people make is thinking they need to make up any hours they missed if they were ill or otherwise unable to participate in their regular jogging routine. This will put extra stress on your knees and calves and should be avoid at all costs. This is true not only of jogging but of any aerobic or resistance exercise routine. The worst thing you can do for your body is to attempt to make up for lost exercise time.

Locating the Perfect Place to Jog

It is important to have a good place to jog, somewhere that is safe and has good, solid ground. You do not want to be on hills or rough terrain because that will be detrimental to your legs and will make it more difficult for you to perform as you would like to do. Trying to jog on a hill at the same time will also cause problems with your jogging routine and could also make it difficult for those who have difficulty climbing hills without jogging. It is important to choose an area that makes it easy to jog, is safe and allows you the opportunity to pace your routine so that you do not have to overexert yourself.

Although it may seem that parks offer a good layout for jogging, you have to make sure you are careful in choosing. If the park is in use as a children's playground, it may not be as level as it should be to make a good jogging trail. In addition, you may find playground equipment that is in the way and will not allow you to jog in a straight line, the preferable means for a good healthy jog. You may also find other rough spots such as rocks and dirt piles that will have a detrimental effect on your routine. In addition, you run the risk of tripping and falling or stumbling while you are jogging. All of these lend way to the possibility of injury.

When looking for the perfect jogging spot you want first to choose an area with a trail that is level and smooth. It will be almost impossible to jog on ground that is rough and uneven. Not only will it make it difficult for you to jog but it may also cause injury to your legs and knees.

If possible, choose a soft surface though not one that is so soft that it inhibits your ability to jog. A track that is customarily used for running is the perfect solution, but you also want to make sure of the surface if there has been a great deal of rain or if it is cold outside. Not everyone is close to a school or college where there is a track, and if they are, it may not be available for the public to use, so you want to choose something that is as close to that environment as possible.

Make Jogging a Group Activity

Quite often, when friends get together they are at a loss for something to do. They have done everything and want something different they have never tried, why not make jogging a group effort? Get some friends together and go for a jog in the neighborhood, the park or the local track. Not only is it a healthy change from going to the ice cream shop but you will be safer in a larger crowd. Although experts recommend at least two people, the more people who are with you when you jog, the safer you will be. By making it a group effort you will be both safe and healthy simultaneously.

Whether you arrange jogging as a group with just friends or participate in a sponsored event is of no relevance. The important issue is taking the time to participate in a group jog with friends or with another group of people. Certainly, it is likely to be more exciting if you are with friends but if that is not possible, do not eliminate the possibility of participating in an activity that is already organized. Do not deny yourself the pleasure of joining in a group jog just because you do not know any of the other participants. Events of this type are the easiest way to meet new people and make new friends.

If you cannot find an event that is already sponsored there is no reason y9ou can't get something started yourself. All you need to do is find a group of people interested in joining in a group jogging activity. You can do it like a game or simply provide healthy refreshments at the end of the job. It is not something that needs a great deal of effort or requires a lot of time to organize. You can send flyers around your neighborhood to let everyone know about the event and see how much interest you can generate. The more people that are interested, the more likely it will be of being successful.

You don't have to participate in a group jogging effort of course, but getting together with a group of friends or others who enjoy jogging can make the time go faster, and you will have accomplished your goal before you realize it. When you make it fun the time goes quickly and you can accomplish more, even beyond the original goals you set for yourself.

Steven Stewart

Protect Your Knees with Proper Shoes

There are special shoes for jogging and other similar exercises. In order to protect your knees you should make certain you wear the proper shoes and that they fit properly. Cross trainers are good for most running and jogging but you may want to ask someone who is experienced in that area if they are right for you. It will depend how much you jog and the kind of ground on which you jog that will make the difference. You do not want to ruin your legs and knees and thus have to give up jogging completely.

Keep in mind that jogging is not good for everyone and for some people simply walking at a brisk pace is the best form of exercise. If you have injured your knees in another activity in the past, you may wish to avoid jogging. The additional pressure to the knees can add additional injury to any you already have. Be safe and be cautious in not only the jogging itself but the shoes you wear when you participate in the activity. Never attempt to jog in regular street shoes or your bare feet. You need the support that is available with sports shoes, preferably one that offers cushioning so you do not come down hard on the balls of your feet and cause damage to your feet.

If you want to continue jogging and even doing other types of exercises that require the use of your feet and knees it's important to make certain you wear proper shoes while you are performing the activity. In addition, if you jog frequently you also want to make sure your shoes fit properly and are in good condition. Most doctors recommend buying new shoes every 8 months—more often if you work on your feet or frequently exercise. No matter how tight your budget may be do not skip on jogging shoes or you run the risk of ruining your feet and your knees. If you have a tight budget look for sales on good shoes rather than skimping and buying jogging shoes that are of a low quality.

For the jogger shoe quality and durability is essential, as is the type of shoe you wear when you are jogging. An ordinary sneaker is not for jogging and will do your feet more harm than good. Consult with a professional in order to choose the shoes that will provide the best protection when you are jogging.

Running or Jogging: the Choice is Yours

Although many people enjoy jogging, others are content with just running or even brisk walking. What is the difference between running and jogging? The major difference is the rhythmic and controlled pace compared to running which tends to have little rhythm to it. While the runner may slow down or even stop every few miles, a jogger tends to go at a steady pace during the entire activity. One of the reasons this may happen is because the jogger maintains a steady slow pace while the runner tends to start out running fast and slows down or stops when he is unable to maintain that pace.

The key is to do what is comfortable for you, but if you want to maintain a regular exercise routine, jogging is better for you than running. That does not mean running is bad but it is more than the short term than the long-term exercise routine. It is more effective to continue at a steady pace instead of changing your pace. This is especially important for those who are unable to run or jog for long periods.

Choosing to maintain an even pace throughout your jogging routine will help you keep your heart rate at the same pace and will prevent you from becoming out of breath or overworked. It is much healthier when you can maintain a steady pace instead of trying to make your heart race and maybe faint or develop cramps.

If you enjoy running and jogging, you may wish to alternate your routine in order to incorporate both of the activities. Keep in mind that you are more likely to last longer during your jogging routine, so save your running for those times you may have less time than others are. Running is a good activity to perform in the morning before you go to work though you may choose a leisurely jog as well.

The important thing is not whether you run or job but to make sure you protect your feet by wearing properly fitting shoes that have a design for jogging. It also means replacing your athletic shoes on a regular basis and not waiting until they are ready for the trash before you do so. Another mistake many people make is to continue jogging when they are experiencing pain in their knees or legs—stop if you are in pain or you will pain a higher price later.

Safety Tips for Joggers

No matter what time you jog or where you go there are important safety tips you should always follow. Although one usually thinks of these as important for women, men can become victims of crimes just as easily as women can. In most cases one thinks that women are victims of rape while men might be subject to muggings but there is no iron clad rules that will define one gender being more or less vulnerable than the other. Your vulnerability depends upon where you go and how you present yourself.

One of the most important safety tips to follow when jogging is to go with a friend. Even during the daylight, it is a good idea to have someone else with you even if it is only to make sure nothing happens to you or to keep an eye out for someone who looks suspicious. Having someone else with you is usually a deterrent to criminals because they do not want to someone else to see them and be able to report the incident. Certainly, there are exceptions to the rule but in most cases; a criminal will not bother someone who is with another person. They do not want to be identified and though they might attempt to attack and kill someone who could be a potential witness, they realize that person may be able to disappear and notify the police quicker than they can attack.

Avoid using a personal stereo when you are jogging, especially at night. Although you may think it helps you keep your pace better when you have music playing, you are also allowing the music to distract you from things that surround you.

You cannot devote your full attention to your surroundings if you have headphones on or ear buds in your ears. Criminals know this and they are always on the lookout for those who do not have their full attention on their surroundings. While you are busy jogging to the music, someone can come out from the bushes, grab you and rape and/or attack you.

Always jog in well-lit and populated areas. It is certainly enticing to jog in the park at night where no one can see you in your sweats or shorts and without your hair and makeup on, but that is very dangerous. Never jog anywhere that you cannot see and hear what is going on around you no matter how safe you may feel. Failure to exercise caution can make you a target for a criminal who may be hiding in the bushes or a dark alley.

Should You Jog when You're Pregnant?

The doctor will tell any pregnant patient to make sure to exercise. However, is jogging an option. The key is whether you were jogging before you got pregnant. Except in rare cases, the doctor will tell a pregnant patient to perform any exercises she performed before she got pregnant but not to start anything new. Of course, that also depends on the weight, age, and health of the mother-to-be, and is something to decide between patient and doctor. There may be any number of reasons a doctor may wish a patient to avoid jogging, so do not assume you can continue to do so without consulting with your doctor first.

Jogging is a very slow rhythmic gait, so in most cases pregnant women can participate as long as their doctor agrees. The farther along you get the more difficult it will become, possibly causing bouncing around of the tummy and thus the baby. Be cautious and sensible when you choose exercise to perform while you are pregnant. Certainly walking is always acceptable, so if you are unable to jog or your doctor does not allow you to do so you can certainly walk. As healthy as jogging is, you do not want to override your doctor and jog if he or she feels you should not do so. No one knows your pregnancy better than your doctor does, so you need to put your faith in those decisions and not assume to know more than the doctor. Remember, it is only for a few months and then you can return to your jogging routine.

Most likely, in the very early stages of pregnancy there is no reason not to participate in jogging. However, as your stomach swells it is less likely you will even feel comfortable attempting to jog. You will have too much of a bulge for it to feel comfortable and will more than likely feel uncomfortable walking let alone jogging. Exercise during pregnancy provides a smoother and easier labor so do not allow being unable to job to deter you from walking. You need to move around and keep limber in order to ascertain you will have an easier delivery. At the same time, you want to choose something that is not going to cause any problems with the baby or your pregnancy thus following your doctor's advice should always be on your agenda for the day.

The Health Benefits of Jogging

Everyone needs to exercise in order to maintain good health. That does not mean you need to spend hours in a gym every week by any means. Some people are not into the gym and for them jogging on a daily basis is the perfect exercise routine. It accomplishes what the exercise intended to accomplish, increase the heart rate and metabolism. Even if your weight is within the normal range, you want to make sure your exercise routine increases the speed of your metabolism so that your weight will remain within the normal range. Of course for those who wish to lose weight there is a need to burn more calories than you consume.

Though it may seem minor to those without a weight problem, exercise is very important. In order to remain healthy you need to exercise enough to increase the heart rate and increase the rate at which your body burns calories. Even without increasing your food intake if you fail to burn off the calories you consume you will begin to gain weight. This is one of the reasons people question why they are not eating any more yet they are gaining weight—a sedentary lifestyle does not leave room for calorie burning.

An added benefit that may not occur to everyone is when you are participating regular in an exercise routine such as jogging you tend to be more conscious of the food you eat. Instead of lying around and munching on chips and other unhealthy foods, you have a greater tendency to choose foods that are good for you. It may be something within the subconscious that makes us do it, but exercise just seems to make us more aware of what we put into our bodies. That is certainly not true of everyone but many people do subconsciously eat better when they take the time to exercise regularly.

How often should you jog? It is a personal decision but if possible, you should jog for at least a half to forty-five minutes every day. If you do not have that much time at once, you can break it into fifteen to twenty minute intervals. Some people use their lunch break to exercise but you have to keep in mind even for short jogs you still need to make certain to wear properly fitting and appropriate shoes in order to avoid damaging your feet, legs and knees.

Using a Track or Jogging Trail

If you are trying to make a decision about whether to jog on an ordinary jogging trail or on a track there are some things to take into consideration. A jogging trail can consist of anything from a park to the sidewalk in your neighborhood. When you look at the difference, it is easy to see which one is preferable. It may also consist of broken sidewalk, hard surface and even hills. All of these will make it very difficult and maybe even create hazards that you do not see before an injury occurs.

A track on the other hand consists or dirt or other soft surface and is within a definite area. You know where to go and the length of the track. You do not have to worry about being lost or out after dark in a remote area on which you have no knowledge. The problem is that many people do not have the convenience of being close to a track or are not able to use the track available. Tracks are most often located on the athletic fields of schools or colleges but they do not always allow the public to use them even for jogging.

Before you begin, a regiment of jogging you may want to decide whether you want to use a track or jogging trail and proceed from there to find a place where you can jog. By choosing your spot before you begin jogging you will have time to locate the right spot for you to perform your activity without having to waste time looking when you get ready to do it. If you anticipate needing more than one location, you want to include that as part of your research as well. Before you begin jogging, you should have several places lined up for your activity.

If you are unsure if you want to use a track or trail, take some time and try both—see which one provides the most comfort. It is always good to take the time to do a "trial run" before you are ready to develop your routine. You want to allow yourself enough time to gather the information you need and discover which options will work better for you. Some people like the softer track while others prefer the firmer trail when they are ready to perform their jogging routine.

Chapter 5- Jog, Sprint and Marathon for Easy Weight Loss

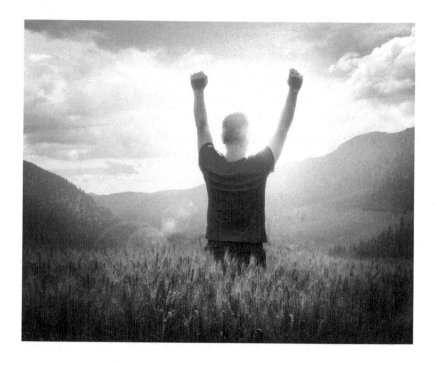

Sprints commonly are tested in track events including 100 m, 200 m or 400 m races. World-class athletes may finish these events in ten seconds, twenty seconds or forty-five seconds, respectively. A marathon is a race that's 26.2 miles long with world-class athletes completing the race in just over 2 hours.

Scientific research has demonstrated that sprinters and marathoners have predominantly different muscle fiber types. Sprinters will have fast-twitch muscle fibers that create greater force and bear a faster contraction or response time. Marathoners have slow-twitch muscle fibers that create force slowly and remain contracted longer.

A big amount of calories and energy are burned during marathons, calling for a significant energy source. To meet this requirement, fat, carbohydrates and protein supply the majority of the energy. Sprinting uses ATP or glucose as energy, as the total amount of energy burned up is lower than in marathons.

Sprinting is an anaerobic activity that lets the muscles contract without oxygen. These anaerobic activities are characterized by short acute bursts of energy utilizing a big percentage of maximal strength. Marathons are an aerobic activity that calls for oxygen to be delivered to the muscles during contractions. Aerobic activities call for a lower level of physical exertion over a longer time period utilizing a lower percentage of maximal strength.

Both sprinting and marathons may provide a number of physical advantages, including weight loss, improved heart and cardiovascular health, expanded strength and endurance and increased bone density. Running likewise may have positive effects on mental health, including treatment of depression or curing addictions.

Should You Sprint?

Sprints are anaerobic, signifying they utilize a different sort of energy than long-distance aerobic actions, and always short. For a lot of individuals, sprints are simply plain fun.

It's exciting to go as fast as you are able to and not have to worry about maintaining the high level of effort for a long time. Sprinting likewise has a lot of applications for daily life, like running for the bus or chasing a toddler.

Although sprinting is a fantastic addition to your workout routine, it shouldn't be the only thing you do.

Sprinting is all about speed. When you center your training routine on one specific element, like speed or strength or endurance, that separate element is going to improve. Integrating sprints into your workout repertoire will make you quicker in 5Ks, marathons, or on the soccer field. Naturally, you can't sustain a sprint pace during a longer run, but you ought to see a decrease in your longer-course times.

Sprinting solely won't help improve your endurance. If you wish to run both faster and longer, mix up your running routine: If you run 4 days a week, do sprints on 2 days and longer runs the other 2 days. Switching things around doubles your benefit and prevents tedium for mind and body.

A study discovered that sprint interval training bettered heart health just as well as traditional endurance training for healthy individuals.

When you exercise at a high intensity, the risk of injury likewise increases. In sprinting, likely injuries include tender muscles, muscle pulls and strains, ankle and knee stress traumas, back issues and, for some individuals, irregular heart rhythms after the exercise.

Exercising at such a high intensity more than 2 days per week won't give your body time to recover totally and therefore increases your chances of injuring yourself. For this reason, it's a great idea to cross-train with a lower-impact, lower-intensity workout like walking or swimming a couple of other days a week.

Finally, whether you decide to sprint comes down to your personal preference. You may love the feeling of putting all your energy into one short, all-or-nothing attempt.

On the other hand, working so hard may wear you out quicker than you like. An extreme novice may not feel comfortable running where others can see her, or may feel like she isn't quick enough.

If your leg muscles aren't strong enough yet, a sprint may make you feel shaky. Or you may just prefer the relaxing, trance-like state that comes with endurance exercise.

Whatever your taste, if you are able to incorporate some high-intensity bursts into your routine, you ought to see improvements in both speed and cardiovascular health.

Sprinting isn't simply a faster version of running. It's almost a different sort of discipline altogether. It calls for the sprinter to learn another body form and form specific muscle fibers. Consequently, sprint workouts likewise must be specifically tailored to train the legs in a really unique way.

Ways To Get Faster

The goal of sprint training is to establish explosive burst, which will let you accelerate rapidly and attain an even greater top speed. This starts with stride length. According to pro sports coaches, your stride length ought to begin at 50 to 60cm near the outset of the race and increase progressively 10 to 15cm every step till you attain an optimum length of 2.3m.

You ought to sprint tall and erect, running on the balls of your feet with a high forward-moving knee drive and extended back leg. As you train, you'll establish fast twitch muscle fibers, which are big muscles that provide quick bursts of energy.

Sprint workouts use short bursts of high-intensity sprint intervals of more than 20m and up to 400 or 600m in length. Every sprint interval is selected from increments of 10m between 20 and 100m and every 50m after that; for example, intervals may be done at lengths of 70m, 80m, 90m, 100m, 150m, 200m, etc. This is fairly similar to high-intensity interval training, but the ultimate goal is quickness instead of sheer physical exercise.

Every day you ought to do a specific number of sets that incorporate several repetitions of short sprints with rests in between. For example, you might choose to do five repetitions of 50m sprints and then three sets of these five repetitions for a sum of 15 50m sprints.

The longer the distance, the fewer sets and repetitions you ought to do. It's possible to construct your own workout, though it's likely more appropriate to follow the structure established by a pro.

There are a lot of variations on the standard sprint workout. Resistance sprints, for example, involve some sort of resistance from a sled, tire or an uphill incline. Aided running is defined as running downhill or with the wind. Intensive tempo calls for running at 75 to 95 percent effort with the aim of building lactic acid. Extensive tempo is similar, but the design is to run slow enough so that there's no buildup of lactic acid.

A former professional sprinter likewise advocates plyometrics, which are exercises especially designed to target and better explosiveness and nervous system response time. Plyometrics are highly dynamic workouts and come in different types, but most of the routine includes some sort of hopping, jumping or skipping.

After all, you wish to improve the ground connection time of your feet. An elite sprinter will make connection with the ground for

0.08 to 0.1 seconds. For an average individual it's about 0.2 seconds. This in turn will better your ability to push off from the ground faster and build even better speed.

Increasing speed endurance lets you work at a higher rate for longer periods. Any athlete who's required to repeat high intensity sprints in prompt succession may benefit from this sort of training. Repetitions and rest intervals are kept short to acquire the ability to tolerate high levels of lactic acid in the muscles. Authorities state that keeping tall and relaxed is the key to success.

Short Sprint

Measure thirty to fifty meters on grass, basketball court, or track. Put a cone at the beginning and at five meter separations. Sprint to the first cone and back. Then, turn and sprint to every cone till you've completed the whole distance. Rest for roughly 90 seconds and then repeat numerous times.

Fartlek Training

Fartlek means "speed play" and was developed in 1937. This workout calls for short bursts of running efforts accompanied by short periods of easy recovery effort. For example, you may run fast for one minute and then recuperate with a slow jog for one minute. Repeat this interval multiple times. A suitable warm-up and cool down are advocated.

Track Intervals

Track intervals are not full-scale runs. They're fast, controlled runs with adequate rest between every repeat. The training advantage happens during the rest interval as the body is presented time to adapt.

The length of the speed intervals deviate depending upon the sport and fitness level of the athlete. Athletes training for a shorter race might do 400 meter repeats with 90 seconds rest period in between every interval. Those training for a longer race might do 1,200 meter repeats with enough rest between each interval.

Cruise Intervals

Like short intervals, measure a short distance between 75 meters to 100 meters. Sprint a short distance and "cruise" to end of the measured out distance. For every repetition, the sprint portion gets longer as the cruise distance lessens. By the last repeat, you'll sprint the whole distance.

CHAPTER 6- DOING YOUR MARATHON RIGHT

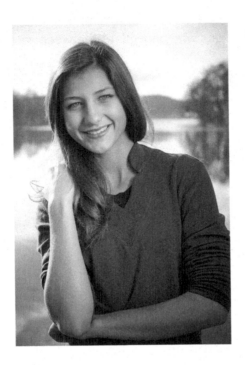

The marathon, over 26.2 miles, is among the most respected athletic accomplishments available to the masses. Anybody may line up in the same event as the best distance runners in the world.

Training for and finishing a marathon call for considerable physical fitness and purpose.

All the same, because marathon running likewise may be an eminently social and even charitable attempt, the sport has exploded in fame, with the number of finishers more than doubling between 1990 and 2010.

Marathon Basics

For you to acquire the satisfaction of completing a marathon, it's vital that you prepare right. Your chances of a gratifying marathon experience that sets you up for a life of running are greater with more running under your belt.

You don't need a wealth of gear to become a serious runner, but because marathoning is an outside and physically stressful activity, you have to be prepared -- particularly when it comes to your feet.

There's no one shoe or group of shoes that's better than the others. A few runners need extra cushioning, a few require a rigid model to control unwanted lateral motion, and others are best-served by a combining of the two.

While select shoes may be found at many outlet stores, you're better off working with learned salespeople at a running specialty store. These shops frequently have discounts on models that have been discontinued but are yet time-tested.

Other crucial issues include how to modify your diet to satisfy your expanded energy needs, which for most individual's means taking in a higher percentage of calories from carbs; increasing your fluid intake; consuming plenty of fiber; and eating littler but more frequent meals.

Center on healthy, colorful foods that help boost the immune system, particularly immediately post-workout -- blueberries with plain yogurt, spinach salad with almonds, red peppers and avocado.

You'll have to pick an appropriate blend of running and walking to begin, and you'll want a running watch as well as a place to keep track of your training advancement.

I advise a run-walk pattern using time, not distance. The opening week may be just twenty minutes of total running time -- for instance, one minute of running and 5 minutes of power walking repeated 6 times every other day. The 2nd week may be 2 and 4, the third three and three, and so forth.

Timing, and not just in the race itself, is everything. Even as you'll need patience and determination to finish the marathon, you'll likewise require them to prepare properly.

Getting your legs and circulatory system used to high-intensity exercise takes time, and mentally adapting to the rigors of an event that consumes anyplace from three to six-plus hours may be as challenging as the physical aspects. If you're heavy or have a chronic medical condition affecting your training, it might take you longer to become set for a marathon.

With the advent of organized marathon-training plans targeting newbies, however, it's no longer rare for individuals to toe the line of a marathon within a couple of months of hitting the pavement for the opening time.

While this is honest for a few, most authorities advise waiting at least a year.

Discovering external support may be a critical factor in your marathon- training success.

When training for a marathon, bearing motivation from partners may make all the difference. Discovering companions who are experienced but evenly matched in fitness is a bonus.

I strongly urge runners to find other people with which to train. It will make each aspect of running better.

Joining a running club likewise may help you meet like-minded souls who have been in your shoes and may help guide you through the frequently daunting process.

Commonly, clubs have specific faster-track workouts scheduled at the same time every week, and these are frequently led by a knowledgeable coach and followed by a bite to eat or additional informal social event.

You Must Breathe Right

Mastering your breathing strategy when running may help you relax and move more fluently. The aim isn't to breathe too deeply or too softly. It's better to find a comfy rhythm that lets you keep your running pace steadfast. As a whole, runners ought to breathe at a rate at which they can't hear their own breathing. Loud breaths mean you're working too hard or breathing too forcefully.

A popular myth about breathing when running is that you ought to breathe in through the nose. While this strategy might help to better your stamina, it's not the most effective way to acquire oxygen into your body.

Rather, when running you ought to breathe in and exhale utilizing your mouth. This both increases the amount of air into the lungs and helps keep your face muscles at ease.

Erratic breathing leads to an erratic running manner. Most pro runners breathe in the so-called "2-2" rhythm. The rhythm works so that you breathe in for 2 strides, then breathe out during the following 2 strides.

You might find that your body better suits a 3-3 or even 4-4 rhythm, but, though the latter is uncommon. During the end of a race you might wish to reduce your exhalation speed to just one step while pressing for the finish line.

Positive end-expiratory pressure -- or PEEP -- may give you a slight increase in oxygen intake when breathing. PEEP happens when you puff your cheeks or tighten your lips when breathing out. This makes it a bit harder for the air to escape.

The pressure keeps the tiny sacks in your lungs that draw oxygen inflated for longer, letting you make more use of every breath. This strategy only applies when you're pushing yourself a bit harder, like running up a steep hill.

Breathing in utilizing your diaphragm and the muscles in your abdomen draws more air into your lungs. A lot of amateur runners breathe utilizing their chest muscles, which brings air into the top of the lungs.

You'll know if you're belly breathing as your stomach will expand as you inhale.

Practice this sort of breathing by lying back on the floor with your hand on your stomach. When you inhale your hand ought to rise and fall back down when you exhale.

CHAPTER 7- CYCLING IS ANOTHER WAY TO DO IT

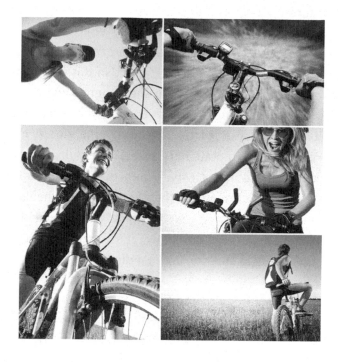

There are many ways to exercise. These experiences range from walking, jogging, swimming to lifting weights, or an assort of other options. You may exercise with any of these. While each accomplishes results when approached seriously, one form of exercise could be added to the list. Many may consider it as a fun activity, but it truly involves exercising. Plus, it is a way to involve inter-generations. It should be no secret. It's bicycling. And, yes, you may exercise for life with this sport.

If you approach the sport as a lifelong experience, you've taken a great leap in several positive directions for yourself. Among the advantages include that you may bike solo, with family members of all ages, with friends or even competitively. In addition, there are opportunities to bike for a good cause. In doing this, you may raise money for that cause, thus helping someone else and yourself at the same time.

Using the term cycling for life, of course, had double meaning. On the one hand, it's a sport that you may enjoy for your entire lifetime. On the other hand, this sport approached through routine exercise may very well extend your life, and in this way makes your life healthier. Who wouldn't want to shed pounds while seeing the world at the same time, even if that world were your own community? Cycling, as a sport, has grown tremendously in the last decade. And, thanks to stationary bikes, depending upon where you live is a year-around activity. When the weather is crummy, your bicycle of choice may be that friendly one-wheeler in the family room or basement. It may not take you around the block, but when it's 32 degrees or below, it's a pretty nice seat for watching the world go by, even it is standing still.

Actually, stationary bikes have several advantages for the person who insists upon taking up more than one task at once. If you can chew up and walk at the same time, chances are pretty good that you can ride a stationary bike and read a book at the same time, or heaven forbid, watch your favorite movie while peddle in your basement. Try that while swimming, jogging or skydiving. You can't do it.

But, as you ride your bike off into the sunset, with the wind at your back, it's a feeling you wouldn't trade for all the weightlifting medals in the world. And the best part is that you may cycle for life no matter what your age or condition of that contraption with two wheels, one chain, a handlebar and a seat.

Bicycle Apparel and Gear

When you ride your bicycle you should consider apparel and gear that will not only bring you comfort but also keep you safe. Consider where you will be riding. What terrain will you be biking through and what is the climate like? Make sure to check the weather before you leave and take the appropriate clothing. Below are some items to consider paying particular attention to in order to make your ride more pleasurable.

When you buy a helmet make sure that it is it approved by the Consumer Product Safety Commission (CPSC) and that it is the right size. Everyone's head it shaped differently so try on different helmets until you find one that is comfortable.

Wear the helmet level on your head and adjust straps and buckles for a proper fit. When you are done adjusting your helmet shake your head to make sure that it does not bounce around. It is one of the most important items that you can purchase and the goal is to protect your head and in turn prevent brain injury.

Some types of apparel and gear to consider are:

• Gloves

• Socks

• Bike shorts

• Jersey

• Jacket

• Shoes

When purchasing rain gear Make sure you are aware of the difference between waterproof and water resistant. To be considered water proof it must be made of water proof fabric and the seams must be sealed. Water resistant is made of material that repels water but is not water proof. Just be aware that there is a huge distinction.

You should always pack up an emergency bike kit. Purchase a small bag that can hook under your bicycle seat. In this bag you should include:

• Tire levers Spare tube

• CO2 Tire inflater Swiss Army knife

• Water bottle to stay hydrated

Drinking enough water is important to many parts of your body, including cells, muscle & joints, brain, kidneys, heart, skin, digestive tract and maintaining your temperature. Even the smallest loss of fluid can affect your concentration and impair your decision making process. Without enough water your body may become overheated and you may not be able to perspire.

Basic first aid

Disposable gloves Antibiotic ointment Sterile dressings Adhesive bandages

If you have special needs such as diabetes makes sure you have you glucose monitor with you and some snacks that will help you remain stable. Follow these simple tips and you too can enjoy cycling for life!

Bicycle Types

There are many types of bicycles to choose from. Which you choose should depend on where you will be riding and what your purpose will be.

Some questions to ask are: Am I riding for pleasure?

Will I be riding for exercise? Will I want to go off road?

How much do I want to spend?

There are touring bikes, utility bikes, mountain bikes and recumbent bicycles, just to name a few. People ride bikes for many reasons. They may use their bike as transportation or just for fun. They can also be used as an exercise tool and for sport. Touring bikes are designed for long trips and have the ability to transport your personal belongings and other gear. These types of bikes are suitable for riding around the countryside and enjoying the view.

Mountain bikes are built to be used off road and have sturdy durable frames and wide-gauge tires. Suspension systems such as gas shocks or air shocks are featured to absorb the impact when on rough terrain.

Recumbent Bicycles are built to maximize comfort and minimize resistance. It may be difficult to get used to being horizontal but if you have any injuries that may prevent you from cycling then you may want to check this type out.

Tandem bikes can be used for those who have some physical challenges. Some considerations are to make sure the bike fits both people. This will help prevent injuries. An important thing to remember is that there can only be one captain.

Downhill biking is usually done on steep terrain. It may not be for everyone.

BMX designed for tricks, stunts and racing on hilly dirt. There are competitions that you can enter and even money to be won.

Single track is a form of mountain biking that is performed on very narrow off road trails that can be steep and narrow with sharp turns and other obstacles. This type of riding takes a lot of upper body strength.

There are bikes that include even the youngest member of the family by attaching a smaller two wheeled bike on the end of a bike.

Ice biking is just what you think it is. People ride through ice and snow. It may not be for everyone because it is more tiring to peddle through the snow.

With all of these choices, no one should be left out.

Chapter 8- Cycling as a Recreational Activity

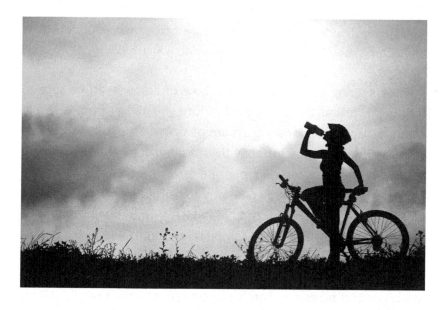

For many who love cycling for life, riding their bikes can be a disappointing experience. While bicycle seats are designed for maximum comfort and efficiency, they are not comfortable for everyone. Many riders experience discomfort while riding or after riding. The shape of the seat can cause soreness or discomfort.

Luckily, there are a number of options for those who love to ride, but who do not love traditional bike seats. First, many recumbent bikes have a different type of seat. If you do not mind the way you have to sit and ride with this type of bike, it is a great option. There are also other types of comfort bikes that work wonderfully.

Additionally, there are special bicycle seats made for people who are made uncomfortable by traditional bicycle seats. There are a few designs that make riding easy while keeping comfort in mind. If traditional bike seats make you uncomfortable, don't worry. You do not have to give up riding because of the discomfort. It is important to continue cycling for life and improving your life, health, and the environment. With a new bicycle or bike seat, you will be able to ride like you love to do and continue exploring.

Whether you ride to work or just ride occasionally for fun, it is important that you are comfortable while you are riding.

If you are going to purchase a new bike or a new seat, be sure to thoroughly test all of your options before you make a choice. While comfort bikes and comfort seats are designed especially for people who are made uncomfortable by traditional bike seats, not all models are perfect for everyone. Be sure the one you choose is perfect for you. The salespeople at your local bike shop should be more than happy to make recommendations and to help you make a selection. They should also completely support you trying out all of your options.

Many comfort bikes are slightly more expensive than regular bikes, but that is not always the case. Depending on the model and design you want, comfort bike seats can range in price from very inexpensive to relatively expensive. Of course, you should be sure to get the bike or bike seat that makes you feel most comfortable, so you can get the most out of your rides.

Biking Accessories Make Cycling for Life Easier

If you are going to cycle for life, you want riding your bike to be as little of a hassle as is possible. A great way to make biking easier is with biking accessories. There are a number of options when it comes to biking accessories, and much of your choice will be based on basic personal preference. However, there are a few accessories that nearly every biker needs to make cycling for life easier.

Some of the most important biking accessories for bikers to have are lights. If you are ever going to bike when it is dark, or getting dark, you must have lights. Depending on the season, it may be dark in the morning or even late afternoon. If you bike to work or for another purpose during these times, lights are essential. Even if you do not plan to bike when it is dark, you should have lights just in case. A solid light is best for the front of your bike, and a blinking light is best for the back of your bike. You may also want to consider reflective clothing if you will be riding at night. It is important to ensure that any car traffic can see you when you are in or near streets.

Another very important bike accessory for safety is a helmet. Helmets are not required in some states, but they are a great choice nonetheless. While you may be a safe rider, it is best to plan for contingencies. A helmet will help protect your head in the event of an accident, no matter what the seriousness. Lives have been saved by bicycle helmets. Besides, there are some modern, comfortable, and stylish designs available.

A tire pump is another great bicycle accessory to have. In the event that your bike tires ever need a bit of air, your tire pump will be a life saver. While it is easy enough to take your bike to a gas station to use the air machine, a tire pump at home will save you time and money. You should fill your tires with an air machine periodically anyway, but it is nice to have a tire pump around if you need it.

Speedometers are a great accessory to have. Many are easy to use, and they can tell you how fast you are riding, and often how far you have gone. Speedometers are a great way to measure your progress during a goal, and are fun to use besides.

Those interested in cycling for life do a lot of good for themselves and everyone else. Health improves, less pollution is made, and they lead by example. In fact, biking has become so popular that easy to use and much needed accessories are surfacing left and right.

While they have been around for a while, bike trailers and cargo bags make cycling for life easier. If you have many things to bring with you, but would like to bike, that is no longer impossible. Thankfully, it is easier than ever to bike with additional belongings. Whether you want to bike to the grocery store and need a place for your grocery bags, or want to bike to a camping locale and need space for your tent and more, biking trailers and cargo bags are just what you need. Biking trailers come with a variety of options.

Traditionally, all the biking trailers seen were for kids. Biking enthusiasts could buckle their children in, and tow them behind their bike. Those are, of course, still available, and much improved. However, there are other biking trailers available today as well. In addition to the traditional child trailers, there are trailers made for storing other items too. These are idea for long rides where you must take luggage of sorts, or even for grocery shopping. The possibilities are endless.

Cargo bags are a smaller and less obvious option than biking trailers. These are ideal for a rider who often struggles with how best to take belongings with them on a ride. Cargo bags are the perfect place to store a briefcase, laptop, files, and a change of clothes if you ride to work. Also, they are perfect for relatively small trips to the grocery store. If you are taking an overnight camping trip, cargo bags can usually hold a small tent and some basic supplies.

How you choose to use your biking trailer and cargo bags to make cycling for life easier is your choice. The options are limitless, and you are sure to find something that works for you and that you enjoy using. With the option of bringing everything you need with you wherever you choose to bike, you might just bike more often, and do more good. The best way to make a choice about a biking trailer or cargo bags is to visit your local bike shop, and browse the options.

Competitive Cycling is a Phenomenon

You probably feel as though you see more cyclists out on the road these days. Not only are people turning to cycling for better health, but they are turning to it as the ultimate rush. Many have looked to cycling as a competitive sport and have reaped the benefits in the process.

Nobody ever used to think of cycling as a legitimately competitive type of sport, but this is the way it is now. It can start with something simple like just one race, and the phenomenon usually starts from there.

What's drawn a lot of people in is that many charity and non-profit groups started sponsoring cycling events to help raise money for their given causes. This pulls at the heart strings of many people and they want to do whatever they can to help. This is where the turning point comes in because once somebody begins with cycling, particularly when it's for a good cause, they're hooked! There are so many great benefits to cycling and when you couple it with the possibility of helping a good cause, it's a no brainer.

Those who sign on to participate in a cycling charity race have no idea how rigorous the training can be. To be able to participate effectively in these races that usually range anywhere from 1-3 days for their completion means months of cycling training and conditioning. It's essential to build up your body, tolerance, and ability to cycle for lengthy periods of time before you can be prepared to participate in the actual race. This is where cycling takes on a different meaning for so many people as they become almost addicted to the way it makes them feel and craves the rush they get from setting out on another cycling path or mission of the day or week.

It's not to say that everybody gets involved in cycling in the same way, but there is definitely a bigger draw to the sport due to so many competitive events rising up. This is great for the non- profits that have money raised for them and excellent for the individuals who get in shape and get drawn into such a rewarding sport. It's really no wonder that as somebody trains for a competitive race; they are quickly pulled into the world of cycling and all it has to offer. This has truly turned into a phenomenon and the good news is that cycling shows no signs of slowing down anytime soon.

Cycling as a Family Activity

It seems that the battle of the bulge has hit just about every age group and walk of life. There is a serious epidemic of childhood obesity happening in this country, and therefore families need to figure out ways to get and stay fit. As many families try to think of attractive ways to get fit together, they often turn to cycling. This is an excellent way to burn some calories, get in shape, and enjoy some family bonding time. So for those families searching for a family activity that will allow them more time with each other and even help them to get in shape, cycling is the answer.

Parents want the best for their children, and when they see that their kids are unhappy or overweight they quickly realize that it's time to do something. The problem with so many types of exercise out there is that they feel too much like exercise and therefore kids won't stick with it.

Cycling however offers something easy to get into, interesting, and presents an excellent opportunity to bond with the family unit as you get fit. This is truly a win-win for many parents as they get to spend some time with their kids and allow them to get in shape in the process. For most kids, cycling doesn't feel like a massive undertaking or an exercise regimen, it is instead something to look forward to as an activity to do with mom and dad.

Cycling can start off rather simply as just a spin around the neighborhood or even around the block if you need to start small. The key to getting kids involved in any activity is to start off slowly and ease them into the physical part of it so that they don't get bored or frustrated.

Cycling can start off slowly and be built up to giving kids some great goal setting potential as they build up their endurance and ability. Once the family overall starts to get in better shape, then it's time to step it up and find some fun routes and paths for the family to travel on. Cycling can quickly become something to look forward to whenever time permits as every time out is a new adventure. The kids can get involved in picking the spots or paths that the family sets out on. You quickly see how cycling can not only become an excellent family bonding activity, but one where the entire family gets in shape without ever feeling like they are exercising.

Cycling as an Excellent Form of Exercise

People never used to look to an activity such as cycling as a robust fitness regimen, but times have changed. Those who used to think that cycling was just a leisurely activity have a lot to learn as this can be one of the most intense and efficient methods of exercise. If you're looking for a good workout, then look no further from cycling as it will help to get you fit and lean rather quickly—it can work wonders when compared to other simpler exercises that you could do in the gym.

Cycling as an excellent form of exercise is definitely something worth looking at, but you just need to log the miles to make it impactful. You get an amazing lower body workout, as well as pulling in the use of your arms, chest, and back as you bike your way to a better body. This is one of those exercises that pulls in every aspect of your body to propel you forward and that is what makes it one of the most comprehensive and effective workouts out there. The world of cycling is changed forever as people quickly realized just how much this form of exercise can create the body that so many are after.

If you log the necessary miles through cycling, you will see the weight literally melt away. You will then see your body start to get toned as you build up muscle in all the right places. You will see the most immediate changes in your legs and lower body overall as these are the muscles working the hardest in cycling. If you are after a toned physique then this is the way to go without a doubt. When it comes to cycling though, you need to be sure that you build up slowly to avoid injury.

Cycling can be exhausting and intense, but well worth it in the long run. You will feel as if you can only go short distances at first, but it's really smart to build up your endurance over time. Cycling can not only help you to look better, but to feel better and certainly will build confidence in the process. So if you have been struggling to find an excellent form of working out but couldn't quite get into something that was effective and fun, then look no further than cycling.

For many, cycling is the most comprehensive and effective exercises out there.

Cycling to Better Health

So many of us are struggling with weight issues or health conditions in some capacity, and something really needs to be done. So when it comes down to getting in shape and feeling better people turn to sports and exercises that they feel comfortable with. This is where cycling comes in as people look to this familiar sport as an easy form of exercise. Most people can benefit from getting healthier and this can contribute to living a longer life that is much more enjoyable. As people start to realize that, they want to find something that will help them to quickly get in shape and still enjoy the activity while they are doing it.

Cycling to better health is a very familiar concept. If you think about it, many of us spent a good many years of our childhood on bikes so the concept is rather familiar and comfortable. This is one of those exercises that doesn't always feel like exercise, though you do need to make a commitment to see the effects. They say that the two best ways to get yourself in better shape and looking the better picture of health is with proper diet and regular exercise. One without the other doesn't work and so along with the healthy eating come the need to exercise. This is the point at which many people turn to cycling as their chosen form of getting fit and feeling better overall.

Cycling can help you to burn major calories, but in a gentle way that doesn't wreak havoc on your body. People of all ages and walks of life can enjoy cycling and that's what makes it so very appealing. You can find some excellent trails outdoors to practice your cycling skills and if the weather turns bad, you can find some excellent options indoors as well. Cycling is very approachable and so for those that wish to gain better health, they turn to this as a starting point. You can perform cycling on your own or with others so it makes it one of those activities that works for just about any situation. If you're looking for an exciting form of exercise or have a vested interest in getting healthier for any number of reasons, then cycling may be just the activity that you have been looking for. Even if you haven't been on a bike for year, cycling can offer a gentle way into the world of exercise and get you feeling better almost immediately.

Cycling for Cardio Health

You truly can cycle for life and improve your cardio health while doing it. Cycling will strengthen heart muscles and is also deemed an excellent cardiovascular exercise. Before beginning any exercise program, check with your doctor. Cycling is a low impact exercise that one can enjoy throughout their life time.

Heart disease can include:

Coronary artery disease Aorta disease

Vascular disease Pericardial disease Heart valve disease Heart failure

Abnormal heart rhythms Congenital heart disease

Prevention: Quit smoking

Lower cholesterol

Control high blood pressure Exercise

The benefits of a good cardio workout are that it builds your endurance and even increases your lung capacity. Endorphins are released and will give you a natural high. You should elevate your heart rate for 20 minutes, break out into a sweat. Vigorous exercise for 45 minutes every other day will be beneficial to your heart.

Exercise is also a stress reliever and we all know that stress affects your heart. There is a link to heart disease and stress. You will always have stress but the trick is to control it and not let it control you. When your stress level rises adrenaline increases your heart rate and blood pressure. Cortisol is a stress hormone is also released and increases sugars in the bloodstream. This in turn changes your immune system, reproductive system and digestive system.

If you do not want to cycle outside, you can sign up for a spinning class at your local gym or buy a stationary bike. The best thing to do is try a spinning class first to see if it is something that you want to do before investing in any equipment.

If you want to ride outside then you should consider visiting your local bicycle shop and getting fitted for a bike that is right for you. You want it to be comfortable and easy to control. Some types of bikes to choose from, depending on what you will be doing are touring bikes, mountain bikes, recumbent bikes, downhill bikes and those that are fitted for wheelchair racing.

Cycling for life is not only a fun sport to take up but is also heart healthy and stress relieving. There are so many benefits that come with cycling. You can include your whole family or go solo. You can ride through the countryside and enjoy the sounds.

CHAPTER 9- PANORAMIC VIEW AND EXTREME WEIGHT LOSS

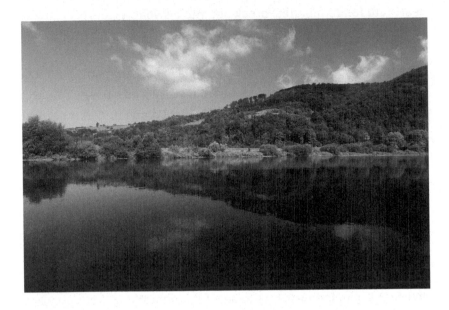

Whether you bike occasionally for fun or enjoy frequently, serious rides, it is good to know the best cities to bike in. Perhaps you have a friend who lives in one, and you need to know if you should bring your bike when you visit. Or, there could be a city near you, or even the one you live in, that you just have to explore.

Portland, Oregon, is often cited as the best biking city in the United States. With rivers, mountains, forests, and other natural wonders around, it is no wonder. Portland is a bike friendly city with bike lanes on many major roads, and even some special roads just for bikes. If you want to commute to work here, it is very easy. Or, if you prefer, it is a great place to take a leisurely ride.

Minneapolis, Minnesota, may be surprising to some. However, when it is not snowing, it is a great place to bike. This twin city is very fun to explore, and a perfect place to bring a bike. Seattle, Washington, is another excellent place to ride your bike. With the

Puget Sound just nearby, you are sure to get an excellent view when you reach the top of a city hill. Even with the notorious northwest wet weather, biking in the fresh air of Seattle is hard to beat.

San Francisco, California, is one of the most unique places in California. What could beat a great view of the gorgeous Golden Gate Bridge, or biking down the most windy road in the world? With new and exciting things to see on every street, it is no wonder San Francisco made the list.

Madison, Wisconsin, is a very bike friendly city, and this does not seem to be changing. In Madison, you can bike around the city or around a lake. The bike routes are marked well and easy for even inexperienced bikers to use.

Austin, Texas, is often compared to Portland, and it is easy to see why. Both of these great cities are on the list of the best places to bike. Austin is bike friendly, and there are so many things to see. You get the benefits of a place like Portland without the pesky northwest rain. Of course, there are many more great cities to bike. In fact, you could make the most of just about any city by biking it. Talk about cycling for life, making a habit out of biking cities is sure to improve your health and the environment!

Great Bike Trails Around the United States

Whether you are a novice biker or an experienced one, you need to know where the great bike trails are. Even if you cannot visit and ride them all, it is possible you will be able to ride some of them. The experience of the greatest bike trails are fantastic, and bikers of all abilities will love them.

In every single state, there are bike trails that are perfect for cycling for life. Some are in urban areas, others are in rural areas. There are a number of bike trails that have been converted from rail road tracks. Some trails are paved, others are dirt or grass. No matter where you live, there are bound to be great bike trails somewhere nearby or at least in your state.

The Okanogan Region of Washington state is on many lists as one of the best biking trails around. In northern Washington, between Spokane and Seattle, is this great place to bike. Fantastic views, wildlife sightings, and fresh air waits.

The driftless area of Wisconsin is in the southern part of the state. This part of the state has hills and valleys that are very fun to ride in. If you are a novice rider, it may be best to wait until you have a higher level of expertise. The ups and downs of riding in this area can make for a tough ride.

Cajun County in Louisiana, offers some fantastic scenic views. Bordering the Gulf of Mexico, there are also swamps, bayous, and more for your viewing and riding pleasure. It can get pretty hot, so be careful of when you choose to visit and ride.

Sugarloaf Moutain in the state of Maryland is a great place to ride for fresh air, views, wildlife sightings, and a cool breeze coming off the water. An added benefit is the relatively close proximity to Washington, D.C.

Finally, Acadia National Park in Maine, has long been a Mecca for bikers. There are so many trails, over one hundred miles worth, that it seems impossible to see everything. This national park allows camping, so it may be best to stay the night and get the full experience.

Wherever you live, there are great places to ride your bike just waiting to be found. Even if your state is not known for being bike friendly, you just have to look for places to ride. Many hiking trails allow bikes, so consider looking into hiking trails if you cannot find many biking trails. Just be sure to confirm that bicycles are allowed.

Cycling for Life By Biking to Work

Biking to work can be a tall order, even for the devoted biker. Given changing weather conditions, time constraints, and more, it is a hard commitment to make. The best way to start biking to work is slowly. Perhaps start with one day per week, and then gradually increase the frequency.

In some places, it just is not feasible to bike to work year round. However, you certainly can bike to work during summer, spring, and at least part of fall in most locations. If you live in a more southern state, you may be able to bike to work all year long.

Biking to work will save you money on gas, which is one of the more obvious benefits. However, it will also save you stress since you do not have to sit in traffic and be stressed.

Also, you will be getting a great deal of exercise that you normally do not get. Even if your job is a mile from your house, if you bike to and from work every day that is ten miles of biking that you would not have had each week. Not only that, but biking instead of driving helps the environment, because the exhaust from your car is not increasing pollution.

If you want to cycle for life, biking to work is one of the very best ways to do it. There are many things you can do to improve your health, and biking to work is a great way to start. The exercise you get while riding you bike to work is very impressive. There are few other ways to get as much exercise and contribute so much to your health on a daily basis. Besides, most people do not have an hour or two each day to spare in order to visit the gym. Instead, add some time to your commute, and work out on your way to work.

It is easy to get a storage basket or bag for your bike, so you can bring a change of clothes with you on your bike, and even a briefcase or backpack. This way, if you get dirty or sweat a bit while riding your bike to work, you can still look clean cut and professional when you arrive, as soon as you change. There are many ways to cycle for life, and biking to work is just one way to start. It is easy to try, and many people live close enough to their place of employment to try it. So don't wait, start cycling for life by biking to work today.

Travel Trips for Cyclers

Cycling is one of those sports that you can learn when you are young and carry on well into your golden years. In fact, you can cycle for life. Do you remember when you received your first bicycle? Did you have training wheels? Remember the excitement when you could ride without them? The thrill of knowing that you can brake and stay upright is one memory that you may never forget.

One of the best things about cycling is that you can do it with your friends or ride alone. You can ride near the oceans, lakes and rivers. There are touring groups that will take you along back roads to see countryside that you would otherwise just pass by if you were in a car.

There are biking trails in many parts of the country now where you can ride through cities as well as the countryside. You can also book a biking trip through many countries and experience unique cultures.

When you are choosing a trip, consider if you want to go on your own or with a guided tour. Guided tours can be fun and safer for you if you are not of an adventurous spirit. The downside of it is that you will have to follow them and not be able to take side trips. Each has its good and bad so make a decision based on what you are comfortable doing.

Use your favorite search engine to find travel options. Some are eco-friendly and include the option of walking and biking which might be something you would be interested in.

Once you decide where you want to go, pay attention to some of these rules of the road:

Headphones should not be worn while cycling Fill medical prescriptions

Make sure you are familiar with all of your equipment

Purchase an extra pair of glasses or contacts or take along your prescription Pay your bills before you leave

Take along a major credit card and/or traveler's checks

Leave a copy of your itinerary with a trusted friend or family member

Above all, make sure you train well before you leave but do not over train so much that you are too tired to enjoy the trip. Maintain a level that will consistent with the geographical area where you will be riding. Ask others who have done this for their suggestions and cycle for life.

Chapter 10- Losing Weight with Your Friends

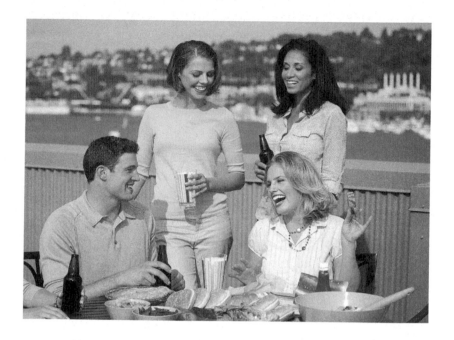

If you are interested in cycling for life, and making the most of cycling, you must look into biking events. Cycling for life can be cycling for others or for yourself, and it is a great way to improve the world around you. You can help the environment, your health, and even raise money and awareness for others.

Many biking events are charitable events, so you can feel good about biking and having a good time. These biking events can make money for a charitable organization in a number of ways. First, they often charge an admittance fee to riders. For example, you may have to pay twenty dollars, but that money is donated to the organization the ride is for. Or, you may need to obtain sponsors who will donate to the organization and support you riding.

More often than not these biking events are relatively long, and often have stops for resting and restrooms. Many times, they will also have obtained corporate sponsorship in products, and will hand out refreshments like water, energy drinks, or energy bars. These donated items are free to riders. Because of this, most of the time you will get back in products the money you paid to ride in the first place, depending on the amount. Biking events like this are similar in many ways to marathons, except you are on a bike instead of running or walking. The length of biking events vary considerably, depending on the purpose of the event and the route.

There are also many biking events that are not for charity, but are just for fun. Depending on where you live, there may be biking events meant to explore the local area, such as riding across all the local bridges or riding up and down a local mountain. Most big cities offer a lot of biking events, and with a little research, you can find the ones that interest you.

Whether you ride in a biking event for charity or for fun, you can rest assured you are still biking for life. After all, the more you bike, the better it is for your health, and the more you are improving yourself. Not only that, but you are encouraging those around you and those who see you riding to ride themselves, which can make a huge environmental impact. Leading by example, in other words, is a surefire way to cycle for life. And riding in a biking event is a great way to make the most of cycling.

Making the Most of Cycling With Organized Bike Rides

More and more people today are interested in improving their lives with cycling. Biking to work, to the store, or just for fresh air and exercise are incredibly common. Biking is also a great way to meet new people and discover things in your area you never knew existed.

A quick internet search can help you find local bikers who are trying to connect with others. If you find a group that bikes together, see about joining them. There are often multiple groups that organize large bike rides and welcome new members. Usually these groups are free.

It is likely that you will be able to find rides that fit into your physical abilities. If you are a relatively new rider, look for a ride that is short and not too strenuous. Most groups have a lot of rides, and you do not have to participate in them all.

Riding with a group can also be safer than riding alone, because your group of bikers will be very visible. Joining an organized bike ride will be fun, interesting, and could even be an educational experience. If you are new to an area, or just new to biking in an area, you will surely discover all sorts of new things. It is highly possible that there are all sorts of neat things in your area you have never seen before. On a bike, you can go many more places than in a car.

If the organized bike ride is large enough, it is possible that some streets will even be shut down, increasing your safety immensely. This is not immensely common for everyday rides, but for big riding events it happens all the time.

If you love to ride your bike, you just have to make the most of cycling with organized bike rides. All you have to do is show up and ride, so it is much easier than planning a route out for yourself. Not only that, but you are sure to meet other riders who very much enjoy riding, so you know you will have something in common with them.

Depending on the length of your organized bike ride, there may be breaks worked into the schedule. This will give you time to rest, use the bathroom, and eat, as needed. Many organized bike rides are just around a local area for an hour or two, and others are of a longer distance and perhaps even overnight. Be sure to pick an organized ride that you feel comfortable with.

My neighbor is into biking like no one else

Could it be that you have a neighbor like mine? He's into biking like no one I know. You might say that he's into cycling for life. And, you know, I'm a bit envious. I believe he's on to something worthwhile. His cycling interests have taken him to points on the map that you've never heard of. He's met scores of interesting people along the way. Plus, his interest in cycling is good for him. His hobby is not only that, it's also a way he keeps physically fit. It's all for fun, but serious, too.

Get him starting talking bicycles and he won't stop. You see, to me a bike has two wheels and chain. Not to my neighbor, who cycling is a lifetime adventure. He can tell the difference between a mountain bike, all-terrain, tandem or kid's bike at 200 yards.

Talk about his cycling knowledge. Whoa. His biking-accessory lingo is like an encyclopedia. We're talking bag, fenders, leg bands, bells, locks, horns, water bottles, racks, mirrors and kickstands. All this time, I thought there was just a basic kickstand. Not so. There's the classic kickstand made from aluminum alloy. He told me that the advantage to this style is that it is lightweight and doesn't corrode. There's the retro top-plate kickstand. It's made for improved clearance. Then, there's the old Z-shape kickstand. It's top plate fits more frames with tighter clearances. And, of course, there's the rear stay-mount kickstands. Prices vary on all these, as you might have guessed.

My neighbor's bicycle interests have helped him stay fit. His weight's dropped from couch potato to slim. He even looks younger and I know that his heart rate is something he could really brag about if he chose to. It's also enabled him to involve his family, on the older end and the younger end of the age spectrum. You see, in cycling, there's a bike for every size, shape and interest level.

One of the nice things about taking up biking for life, as in my neighbor's case, is that you can start with a pretty basic bike. I've seen him hand down last year's bike to a younger family member, while he moved up from a basic 10-speed to a 27-speed. Yikes. Not to worry, he says shifting gears is like, well riding a bike. Funny thing, he's now got me hooked. The last time he upgraded bikes, he offered me a deal on what might have been his trade it. You know what? I'm bike and enjoying it, too. You might even say that I've taken up cycling for life. I've already dropped one inch around the belt. Who's complaining? Not me.

The Cycling Vacation

Many people are looking for alternative vacation types these days. Either because of tough financial times or the necessity for a more creative type of getaway, people are looking for alternatives that can offer excitement and a more budget friendly option. This is about the time that many people turn to cycling as a vacation option.

The beauty of a cycling vacation is that it involves some great physical activity and also a way of checking out the scenery in the places you visit. Cycling offers all the various aspects of what people look for in a vacation and therefore has become a very popular activity to center a vacation around.

A cycling vacation can take place anywhere. It can be on a campground, at a national park, or as part of a bigger vacation. All it takes is a bicycle and some perseverance to check out the local scenery and take in some new trails. This is appealing for the individual or family who wants to stay fit even on vacation, or for those that wish to see every inch of the place they travel to. Cycling is a friendly activity as it appeals to people of all ages, and therefore makes it approachable and fun. There are even some places out there that offer no motorized vehicles within their perimeters, allowing only bicycles. This is the perfect venue for those that want to check out the beauty of nature and get back to a more simplistic way of living. This is the basis of a great cycling vacation and makes many people seek these vacations out quite often these days.

Cycling as a vacation option never used to be quite so popular, but then again the sport has gained some major attention lately. Couple the increase in popularity of this sport with the fact that people need to take more cost effective vacations in tough economic times and you find that a cycling vacation is truly a slam dunk for everyone. If you are willing to take a more adventurous route for your vacation needs, and you want to get fit in the process, then this is definitely an excellent option. If you have never considered a cycling vacation, then now may be the time. You can find some great destinations, trails, and visit some really great places in the process. To see the land and get in some exercise in the process, a cycling vacation helps you to accomplish it all.

No mud puddles to worry about on this bike

Today, persons are exercising at nearly any age. While the older one gets, the choices may appear to be limiting. One exercise choice for persons of any age is bicycling. In fact, cycling for life is an option that many persons entering their senior years have chosen in keeping fit.

Say you've reached your fourth decade or even higher. You aren't as fit as you once were, but you still want to work up a good sweat and feel in control of things. There are still several options for exercise. Among them is swimming, jogging, low-impact aerobics, and, yes, biking. For the 40-year-old, or older, for example, biking becomes a good exercise option, especially for persons with osteoarthritis of the knees. And the best answer for a knee problem may be a stationary bike.

The good news is that stationary bikes come in many forms. For example, there's the upright stationary bike. It's perhaps the most common stationary bike that comes to your mind. It resembles a street bike, except that gears replace its wheels. The good thing about uprights is that they don't require much space. They feel very natural, especially to the biker who really wishes to be out on the road. In addition, some upright bike exercisers claim that they obtain a better workout than riding on the street. That's because on a stationary bike there is more effort placed into the ride.

Another stationary bike option is the recumbent stationary bike. It's especially helpful for persons with balance or back problems. These bikes also offer more padding. In many cases, recumbent stationary bikes may be easier to ride and read or watch TV during the workout.

While comparing stationary bikes, don't forget about the dual-action stationary machine. It combines upright exercise with movable handlebars. This option gives the rider's arms a real workout. While many stationary bikes boast lower-body workouts, the dual-action bike offers better all-around total fitness. Usually these bikes cost more and are often larger than other stationary bikes.

So, if cycling for life is your thing, but age is a barrier, a stationary bike may be the answer. Workouts on stationary bikes are low-impact; yet enable the biker to burn lots of calories. Perhaps the best feature of a stationary bike is that the chances of hitting an unexpected mud puddle are slim to none. It's not a bad way to spend an hour or so while exercising.

Let me guess. You'd really like to take up an exercise program. You'd like to do something that, well, puts that exercise guru neighbor of yours in the dust, so to speak. You know the neighbor. The slim one who belongs to the fitness club. In addition, for reasons you can't explain, this neighbor always looks healthy, probably because whatever exercise routine is followed is done with meticulous care.

So, where does that put you? Here's a thought. How about checking all those two-wheeled objects in your garage. You know the ones. They come equipped with a seat, handle bars and a reflector or two. Sadly, they also include cobwebs from lack of use. It's a sad site, you and those objects. Let's call them bicycles built for you. The beauty of those sleek machines is that with some effort you might become the envy of every exercise queen or king living next door.

Beyond that, age doesn't matter. Cycling could, in fact, be the thing for you. The best part is you already know how to ride. The most difficult part may be hauling the bike down from its storage area on the garage wall to the floor, where it belongs. Actually, it belongs on the road with you and your bike helmet heading north.

Go ahead; there it hangs like a forgotten trophy. Pretty sad, isn't it. But, using the even sadder cliché, "Today is the first day of the rest of your life," might be all that's needed. Simply get on that bike and change your life. Cycle for the rest of your life. Here's some advice for those just starting out. Think of cycling as a hobby and as an exercise experience, because that's exactly what it is. Beyond that, just to play it safe, take your cycling machine to your nearby bicycle shop. It may need a good going over before you launch into a five-mile venture.

You'll happily discover that the bicycle repair guy treats most two-wheelers like a kid with a new puppy. He'll check your brakes, seat, hand bars, tires, chain and reflectors. Did we miss anything? Once you get the repair shop's green light, head for the hills, baby. Remember, there are always two sides to the hill ahead. One way goes up, but the other goes down. Cycling for life is sort of like the stock market in that sense. What other sport can you name that offers peaks and valleys. Only, unlike the stock market, it's much more fun going down that up.

The Health Benefits of Cycling for Life

There are so many health benefits to cycling for life, it is almost impossible to enumerate them. As such, only a few will be explored. Everyone knows that biking is a great way to improve health, but it is important to know just how good biking is for you.

Biking is one of the best types of exercise, for a number of reasons. First, for many people, it is easier to burn calories on a bike than doing another activity. The reason for this varies person to person, but many people agree it is because biking is so fun. Also, it is easy to do. There is even a saying about how people never forget how to ride a bike. Even if you have not ridden a bike in years, chances are you still know how.

A great health benefit of cycling for life is that your metabolism will increase. Exercising in general jump starts your metabolism, allowing you to burn more fat and calories. With an increased metabolism, it will be easier for you to reach any health goals you may have, or even a target weight if you want to shed pounds.

With a higher metabolism and regular exercise on your bike, you will start to burn fat. Even if you do not necessarily want to lose weight, burning fat is good. Most people have a higher percentage of body fat than they should, and burning that fat helps keep you healthier.

While burning fat on your bike, you will also be building muscle. Riding a bike is an activity that utilizes mostly your lower body, but it does work your core and your upper body a little as well. Building muscle will help give you a healthy look, feel better, and be stronger. It is unlikely that you will build more muscle than is healthy or than you would like if you are not trying to do so, so do not worry about that.

Biking also helps you keep up your endurance or stamina, especially when you bike as a cardiovascular activity. It is important for your overall health that you increase your heart rate while exercising. While you may not want to bike rapidly for your entire ride, perhaps doing so for a mile or two will be a big help to your health.

Finally, exercising has been said to increase your overall level of happiness. Of course, getting fresh air while you go for a ride is sure to elevate your mood anyway. With both physical and mental benefits, cycling for life seems like a great choice.

The Environmental Benefits of Cycling for Life

If you are considering becoming a biker, or if you already are a biker, you know there are a number of benefits to cycling for life. You can improve your own health, the health of those around you by leading by example, and even the world around you by helping the environment. While helping the environment can seem like an astronomical task, it is possible to affect positive change with small steps. You likely already to a number of great things, such as recycle or reuse containers. Cycling for life is just one more step you can take to ensure the world becomes a better, healthier place.

When you bike instead of drive in your everyday life, you do a great deal of good for the environment around you. For example, you are helping the noise level on your commuting route to decrease. If your vehicle is not driving its normal route, it is not making noise. This decreased noise level helps the areas you drive through and around to become more livable communities. While it may seem as if just one car missing from your commute route will make a difference, the fact is that it will.

You may not notice, but it does have an impact. An in influencing others to bike like you do, you will be decreasing the noise level even more. Of course, one of the most obvious environmental benefits of cycling for life is pollution. Even cars that boast great gas mileage give off pollution in their exhaust. If you bike instead of drive, you are helping to decrease car emissions, which helps less greenhouse gases develop. Perhaps you do not want to bike to work each day. If you bike to work even one day a week or month, your actions will have great consequences. If every single person biked to work only one day a week or month, the environmental benefits are almost unimaginable.

Finally, leading by example is an environmental benefit of cycling for life in and of itself. If you inspire even one person to bike occasionally instead of drive, you are impacting noise level and pollution levels even more. Even if you do not convince someone outright to bike, somebody may watch you ride passed them on your way to work each day, and that will help convince them to do the same.

ABOUT THE AUTHOR

Healthy lifestyle is the key to happy, successful and longer life. This is the very principle of the author of this book, Mr. Steven Stewart. Steven is a certified nutritionist. He and his brother are dedicated to help youth to middle-aged people create awareness of the long list of benefits for having a healthy lifestyle.

Aside from jogging and cycling, Steven is also a freelance financial consultant in the city of New York.

CPSIA information can be obtained
at www.ICGtesting.com
Printed in the USA
LVOW01s1518120716

496013LV00009B/38/P